Table of Contents

Hypoglycemia is a condition in which your blood sugar (glucose) level is lower than the standard range. Glucose is your body's main energy source.

Hypoglycemia is often related to diabetes treatment. But other drugs and a variety of conditions — many rare — can cause low blood sugar in people who don't have diabetes.

Hypoglycemia needs immediate treatment. For many people, a fasting blood sugar of 70 milligrams per deciliter (mg/dL), or 3.9 millimoles per liter (mmol/L), or below should serve as an alert for hypoglycemia. But your numbers might be different. Ask your health care provider.

Treatment involves quickly getting your blood sugar back to within the standard range either with a high-sugar food or drink or with medication. Long-term treatment requires identifying and treating the cause of hypoglycemia.

BREAKFAST

1. Skillet Breakfast Potatoes

Prep Time: 10 Minutes

Cook Time: 10 Minutes

Servings: 2

Ingredients

- 2 slices thick-cut bacon
- 3 Yukon Gold potatoes, scrubbed and diced (about 2 cups)
- 1/4 cup finely diced onions
- 1 teaspoon freshly minced garlic
- 1/4 teaspoon salt or to taste
- 1/8 teaspoon freshly cracked black pepper or to taste
- 1/2 tablespoon unsalted butter
- 4 eggs, drained
- Salt & pepper to taste
- 1 cup fresh baby spinach

Instructions

1. Fry up 2 slices of thick-cut bacon in a cast-iron skillet over mid-high heat until just a little crispy. This will only take about 2 minutes, total, but that time will vary depending on how crisp you like the bacon and how hot your pan is. I cut my bacon slices in half to fit in the pan better.

2. While the bacon is cooking, dice up 2-3 Yukon gold potatoes so you have about 2 cups of diced potatoes.

3. When the bacon is crisped to your liking, remove it from the skillet and drain on paper towels. When the bacon is cooled, crumble it and reserve until needed.

4. Add the diced potatoes to the hot bacon drippings in the skillet set over mid-high heat. Spread the potatoes out to a single layer the best you can and then WALK AWAY! Set your timer for 3 minutes and STEP AWAY FROM THE POTATOES! Put down that spatula! There should be NO stirring of the potatoes until they get a nice crispy edge on the one side.

5. When the timer goes off, check to make sure there is a nice crispy crust on the potatoes by lifting one or two of them up. If you see a gorgeous golden and crispy bottom on your test pieces then you have the green

light to gently start turning those potato cubes over. Carefully stir them around in the pan trying to flip them over the best you can. Don't worry if you don't get all of them perfectly flipped over.

6. Reduce the heat to mid-low, add 1/4 cup diced onions and 1 teaspoon garlic. Sprinkle with 1/4 teaspoon kosher salt and 1/8 teaspoon freshly cracked black pepper. Continue to cook the potatoes until they are softened to your liking.

7. While the potatoes are cooking, heat a non-stick skillet over mid-high heat and melt a 1/2 tablespoon of unsalted butter. Carefully crack an egg into a fine mesh strainer set over a bowl to drain out the thin egg whites. The very thin egg white always cooks up too crispy to my liking, so I prefer to drain it first before cooking. It results in a better looking and tasting fried egg, in my opinion, and doesn't take but a few extra seconds. Totally worth it!

8. After draining the thin eggs whites, carefully pour the remaining egg into the hot butter in the skillet. Repeat this process with the remaining eggs. Allow to cook for 3-4 minutes until the eggs are cooked how you like. Mine usually takes a good 3 minutes, but the time will vary depending on the heat of your skillet

and how cooked you like your eggs. I like mine to still have a soft egg yolk when I cut into it. The drippy egg yolk adds a nice flavor to the overall dish. Finish it up by seasoning the eggs with salt and pepper. You can fry multiple eggs at the same time in this manner depending on the size of your skillet.

9. While the eggs are cooking, give the potatoes a little stir now and then and when they are soft the way you like them, turn off the heat, and add a cup of fresh baby spinach (or more to your liking). Wilt the spinach slightly and give the potatoes a taste. Adjust the seasoning as needed.

10. Divide the potatoes onto serving plates and top with eggs. Sprinkle with the reserved bacon and enjoy!

Prep Time: 5 Minutes

Cook Time: 10 Minutes

Servings: 1

Ingredients

- 3 slices thick cut bacon
- 1/2 cup Swerve Sweetener
- 1/2 tablespoon cornstarch
- 1/4 teaspoon salt
- 1/4 cup white vinegar
- 2 tablespoons water
- 2 cups fresh baby spinach leaves
- 1 tablespoon freshly grated cheddar cheese
- 1/2 tablespoon unsalted butter
- 2 eggs
- salt and pepper to taste

Instructions

1. To make the dressing, fry up 3 thick cut slices of bacon in a skillet. I cut my bacon in half to fit a little

easier in the skillet. When cooked to your liking, remove it from the skillet and drain on paper towels to cool and then crumble it. Leave the bacon grease in the skillet.

2. Whisk together 1/2 cup Swerve, 1/2 tablespoon cornstarch, and a 1/4 teaspoon kosher salt. Pour in 1/4 cup white vinegar and 2 tablespoons water and whisk to combine. Pour the Swerve mixture into the skillet with the bacon drippings and heat over medium, whisking until thickened. Give it a taste and adjust the flavor as needed. Add more Swerve if you prefer it sweeter or more vinegar if you like it a little more tangy. Add 1/4 cup of crumbled bacon pieces and stir to combine. Give it a taste again and add salt and pepper to your liking. Drizzle over 2 cups of baby spinach leaves and toss to coat and sprinkle with some freshly shredded cheddar cheese. NOTE: Reserve remaining bacon pieces for another use or sprinkle on top for an extra bacony treat .

3. Heat a non-stick skillet over mid-high heat and melt a 1/2 tablespoon of unsalted butter. Carefully crack an egg into a fine mesh strainer set over a bowl to drain out the thin egg whites. The very thin egg white always cook up too crispy to my liking, so I prefer to

drain it first before cooking. It results in a better looking and tasting fried egg, in my opinion, and doesn't take but a few extra seconds. Totally worth it!

4. Carefully pour the remaining egg into the hot butter in the skillet. Allow to cook for 3-4 minutes until the egg is cooked how you like it. Mine usually takes a good 3 minutes, but the time will vary depending on the heat of your skillet and how cooked you like it. I like mine to still have a soft egg yolk when I cut into it. The drippy egg yolk adds a nice flavor to the overall dish. Finish it up by seasoning the egg with salt and pepper. You can fry multiple eggs at the same time in this manner depending on the size of your skillet.

5. When the eggs are done to your liking, place them on top of the salad and drizzle on some more bacon dressing if you like. Enjoy!

Prep Time: 10 Minutes

Cook Time: 10 Minutes

Servings: 4

Ingredients

- 2 tablespoons butter
- 2 apples, peeled, cored and sliced thinly
- 1 teaspoon cornstarch
- 1/4 cup water
- 1/4 cup brown sugar
- 1/2 teaspoon ground cinnamon
- salt to taste
- 6 large eggs
- 1/4 cup milk
- 1 teaspoon cinnamon
- 1/2 teaspoon vanilla
- 1 tablespoon sugar
- Cinnamon Swirl Bread, day old stale bread work best
- Ghee for cooking the french toast in the skillet

Instructions

1. Melt 2 tablespoons butter in a large skillet over mid-high heat. Add the apples and cook, stirring, until apples are almost tender. About 5 minutes or so.

2. Dissolve 1 teaspoon cornstarch in 1/4 cup water and add this mixture to the skillet with the apples. Stir in 1/4 cup brown sugar and 1/2 teaspoon cinnamon. Add a pinch of salt and bring to a boil until thickened. This should only take a minute or 2. Give it a taste and add more salt, sugar, and/or cinnamon to your liking. Remove from heat and set aside until ready to use.

3. Whisk together 6 eggs and 1/4 cup milk. Add 1 teaspoon cinnamon, 1/2 teaspoon vanilla, and a tablespoon of sugar. Whisk until combine well.

4. Heat a skillet over medium heat and lightly grease with ghee. Dip bread slices in egg mixture and place in skillet in a single layer. Cook bread about 2-3 minutes on each side until golden brown. Repeat with remaining egg mixture.

5. Serve French Toast topped with the sauteed apples and maple syrup. Enjoy!

Prep Time: 10 Minutes

Cook Time: 20 Minutes

Servings: 4

Ingredients

French Toast:

- 1 loaf Brioche or Challah bread
- 5 eggs, large
- 1 1/2 cups heavy whipping cream or whole milk
- 2 tsp cinnamon
- 4 tbsp butter or ghee, divided

Bananas Foster Topping

- 1 cup Pecans, chopped
- 1 cup Maple syrup
- 1/2 cup Brown sugar
- 1 tsp Rum extract
- 1 pinch salt
- 4 Ripe bananas, sliced

Instructions

French Toast:

1. Crack 5 eggs and add them to a mixing bowl. Whisk them together. Add 1 1/2 cups heavy whipping cream (or whole milk) and 2 tsp. cinnamon to the eggs. Mix together completely.
2. Pour the egg mixture into a shallow dish. Place as many pieces of brioche or challah bread as will fit into the dish. Turn them over to completely coat on both sides.
3. Heat a skillet or griddle to medium low. Add a pat of butter and completely coat the surface with the butter (can also use oil and butter or ghee). Place as many pieces of the coated bread in the pan and toast for 3-4 minutes on each side or until they are lightly golden. Remove the French toast from the skillet and keep warm.
4. Coat another batch of bread in the egg mixture. Place another pat of butter in the pan and coat the surface. Toast the second batch of bread and repeat this process until the whole loaf is toasted.
5. Bananas Foster Topping:

6. Heat a skillet to medium low. Add 1 cup of chopped pecans to the skillet. Toast for 5 minutes or so, stirring occasionally.

7. Add 1 cup of maple syrup and 1/2 packed cup brown sugar to the skillet. Bring the heat to medium and stir the mixture together.

8. Slice 4 bananas and add them to the skillet along with 1 tsp. rum extract and a pinch of salt. Allow the mixture to simmer for another 2 minutes or so. Make sure all the bananas are coated in the syrup and slightly caramelized.

9. Serve the French toast. Spoon as much or as little of the syrup mixture over the French toast as you like.

Prep Time: 10 Minutes

Cook Time: 4hrs 20 Minutes

Servings: 4

Ingredients

- 1 loaf bread diced (stale works great)
- 6 eggs
- 2 cups milk Dairy Free Alternative can be used
- 1/2 tsp cinnamon
- Topping
- 1/4 cup butter or Dairy Free Margarine Softened
- 1/2 cup firmly packed brown sugar
- 1 tsp cinnamon
- 1/2 cup chopped pecans
- Dash of nutmeg

Instructions

1. Whisk together eggs, milk and cinnamon and pour over diced bread in a large bowl. Cover an let it soak overnight in the fridge or atleast 4 hours.

2. When ready to bake spray the inside of the crockpot (4-6 quart sized works best) to avoid sticking.

3. Pour in Bread Mix.

4. In a small bowl mix together butter, brown sugar cinnamon, pecans and nutmeg.

5. Crumble of the top of the bread mix. Cover and Cook on low for 4 hours...or if you are in a hurry High for 2 hours.

6. Let sit for 15-20 minutes and serve!

Prep Time: 10 Minutes

Cook Time: 2hrs 20 Minutes

Servings: 2

Ingredients

- 5 cups old-fashioned rolled oats You can use Gluten Free
- 1/2 cup ground flaxseed optional
- 3/4 cup coconut oil or butter
- 3/4 cup honey
- 2 Tablespoons vanilla extract
- 2 Tablespoons cinnamon
- 1 1/2 cups unsweetened shredded coconut
- 1 cup chopped nuts of your choice
- 1 to 2 cups dried fruit chocolate chips, or other mix-in of your choice

Instructions

1. In a small saucepan, melt the coconut oil (or butter). Once it has turned into a liquid, mix in the honey to form your sauce.
2. Mix Oats, Flaxseed, nuts and cinnamon in your crockpot. Add the honey mixture as well as the vanilla and cinnamon. Stir thoroughly.
3. Allow the granola to cook on low for 2-4 hours. You may want to stir every hour to avoid burning. You are also going to leave the lid cracked a little to allow the moisture to escape.
4. Cooking times will greatly vary depending on your crock pot as they all cook at slightly different temps.
5. Allow to cool, then mix in the dried fruit and/or chocolate chips. Store in the refrigerator in an air-tight container for several weeks.

Prep Time: 10 Minutes

Cook Time: 10 Minutes

Servings: 4

Ingredients

- 8 eggs
- 1 tablespoon milk
- 1 tablespoon butter
- ¼ cup finely diced bell pepper
- 2 green onions sliced, whites and greens divided
- 1 cup sharp cheddar cheese
- 6 slices bacon cooked and crumbled
- 8 small corn or flour tortillas warmed
- ¼ cup sour cream
- ¼ cup salsa

Instructions

1. Whisk eggs and milk with salt and pepper to taste.
2. Heat tortillas according to package directions. Wrap in foil to keep warm.

3. Melt butter in a non-stick skillet over medium heat.
    Add the whites of the green onions and the bell
    peppers. Cook until tender, about 3 minutes.
4. Add eggs and scramble until set but still shiny.
5. Divide eggs over tortillas. Sprinkle cheese over top
    and cover for 1 minute to allow cheese to melt (or
    broil 1 minute if desired).
6. Top with crumbled bacon, sour cream, salsa and
    desired toppings.
7. Serve immediately.

Prep Time: 45 Minutes

Cook Time: 15 Minutes

Servings: 6

Ingredients

- 2 pounds Yukon gold potatoes ½ inch pieces
- 1 pound chorizo sausage casing removed
- 4 strips bacon sliced
- 1 onion diced
- 4 cloves garlic minced
- 1 teaspoon coriander
- 1 teaspoon cumin
- ¾ teaspoon smoked paprika
- 6 eggs whisked
- 1 cup cheddar cheese shredded

Instructions

1. Preheat the oven to 375°F.

2. Place the potatoes in a large pot with 6 cups of water, bring to a boil and cook for 6-8 minutes or until they are fork tender. Drain them and set aside.

3. While potatoes are cooking, heat a large skillet over medium heat. Cook the bacon until crisp. Remove and set aside.

4. Remove the casing from the chorizo and add it to the bacon fat along with the onion. Cook until no pink remains, about 8 minutes. Remove from the pan and set aside leaving the fat in the pan.

5. Turn the heat up to medium high and add the potatoes, seasonings, and garlic to the pan. Cook until browned without stirring too much so the potatoes can form a crust. Stir in the meat.

6. While potatoes are browning, lightly scramble the eggs in a small pan over medium heat. Eggs should be slightly undercooked and shiny. Place on top of the hash and sprinkle cheese on top.

7. Place in the oven and heat until cheese is melted and heat through, about 5 minutes.

Prep Time: 10 Minutes

Cook Time: 1hrs 15 Minutes

Servings: 6

Ingredients

- ½ pound sausage crumbled
- ½ cup red or green peppers diced
- 6 cups bread cubes slightly dried
- 2 cups cheddar cheese shredded, divided

Egg mixture:

- 4 eggs
- 1 ½ cups milk
- ½ cup light cream or half and half
- ½ teaspoon dry mustard powder
- ½ teaspoon salt
- ¼ teaspoon pepper
- ¼ teaspoon onion powder

Instructions

1. Preheat oven to 350°F.

2. Cook sausage over medium heat until no pink remains, drain the fat and return the sausage to the pan. Add the peppers and cook until partially tender. Set aside to cool.

3. Whisk the egg mixture in a bowl. Add bread, peppers, sausage, and half of the cheese. Toss to combine. Let sit for 5 minutes and toss again until the liquid is absorbed.

4. Add the mixture to a greased 2 qt baking dish. Refrigerate at least 30 minutes or up to 24 hours.

5. Cover and bake for 30 minutes. Uncover, top with remaining cheese and bake an additional 15-20 minutes or until set in the middle.

6. Rest 10 minutes before cutting.

Prep Time: 20 Minutes

Cook Time: 1hrs 15 Minutes

Servings: 8

Ingredients

- 12 slices cinnamon bread cut into 1-inch cubes, about 12 cups
- 1 cup carrots shredded
- ⅔ cup crushed pineapple drained and squeezed very dry
- ½ cup raisins
- 8 eggs
- 2 cups milk
- ⅓ cup brown sugar
- 1 teaspoon cinnamon
- cream cheese mixture
- 8 ounces cream cheese room temperature
- ¼ cup sugar
- 1 teaspoon orange zest

Topping:

- ¼ cup chopped pecans
- 2 tablespoons butter
- 2 tablespoons flour
- 2 tablespoons flaked coconut
- 1 tablespoon brown sugar
- ½ teaspoon cinnamon

Instructions

1. Leave your bread out for a few hours or place it on a tray at 350°F for about 8 minutes to slightly dry it out.
2. In a medium bowl, combine cream cheese mixture ingredients until fluffy.
3. Grease a 9x13 inch baking dish. Layer half of the bread cubes in the pan. Sprinkle with half of the carrots, pineapple and raisins. Dot with the cream cheese mixture. Top with remaining bread and the other half of the carrots, pineapple, and raisins.
4. In a bowl, stir together the eggs, milk, brown sugar, and cinnamon. Pour over the casserole, cover with foil and refrigerate overnight.
5. Remove the casserole from the fridge about 45-60 minutes before baking. Preheat the oven to 350°F.

6. Mix topping ingredients together in a small bowl. Sprinkle over casserole just before baking.

7. Bake uncovered 45-55 minutes or until a knife inserted in the center comes out clean and casserole is set.

8. Cool 15 minutes before serving.

Prep Time: 10 Minutes

Cook Time: 20 Minutes

Servings: 4

Ingredients

- 2 tablespoons olive oil
- ½ cup onion diced
- 4 cups frozen hash browns thawed
- 1 ½ cups leftover ham diced
- ½ green pepper finely diced
- 4 eggs
- salt and pepper to taste
- ¼ cup cheddar cheese shredded

Instructions

1. Preheat oven to 375°F.
2. Heat olive oil in an ovenproof skillet over medium heat. Add onion and cook until softened, about 5 minutes.

3. Stir in hash browns, ham, and green peppers. Cook until the hashbrowns are lightly browned, stirring occasionally.

4. Press the back of a spoon into the hashbrowns to create 4 wells. Crack a fresh egg into each well. Season with salt and pepper and top with cheese.

5. Bake for 12-15 minutes or until the eggs are cooked to your preference. *Note, the eggs will continue to cook once removed from the oven so do not overcook.

11. Mini Chicken Quesadillas

Prep Time: 20 Minutes

Cook Time: 10 Minutes

Servings: 8

Ingredients

- 1 1/2 cups leftover finely shredded rotisserie chicken
- 1 1/2 cups shredded Mexican blend cheese
- 1/3 cup restaurant-style salsa
- 1/4 cup chopped fresh cilantro leaves
- salt and freshly ground black pepper, to taste
- 1 cup refried beans, homemade or store-bought
- 16 street tacos flour tortillas
- 3 tablespoons canola oil, divided

For Serving:

- 1 cup guacamole
- 1 cup pico de gallo
- 1/4 cup sour cream

Instructions

1. Preheat oven to 200 degrees F.
2. CHICKEN MIXTURE: In a medium bowl, combine chicken, cheese, salsa and cilantro; season with salt and pepper, to taste.
3. Spread refried beans on half of the tortilla; top with CHICKEN MIXTURE, folding over to seal. Repeat with remaining tortillas to make 16 quesadillas.
4. Heat 1 tablespoon canola oil in a large cast iron skillet over medium low heat. Working in batches, add quesadillas to the skillet in a single layer and cook until golden brown, about 1-2 minutes per side; keep warm in oven up to 30 minutes. Repeat with remaining canola oil and quesadillas.
5. Serve immediately with desired toppings.

Prep Time: 35 Minutes

Cook Time: 55 Minutes

Servings: 4

Ingredients

- 8 ounces Barilla fettuccine pasta
- 4 tablespoons unsalted butter, divided
- 2 boneless, skinless chicken breasts
- 1 teaspoon Italian seasoning
- salt and freshly ground black pepper
- 4 cloves garlic, minced
- 1 1/2 tablespoons all-purpose flour
- 1 tablespoon tomato paste
- 1 teaspoon dried basil
- 1 3/4 cups 2% milk
- 1/2 cup finely chopped sun-dried tomatoes
- 3 ounces reduced fat cream cheese, cubed
- 1/2 cup freshly grated Parmesan
- 2 tablespoons chopped fresh parsley leaves

Instructions

1. In a large pot of boiling salted water, cook pasta according to package instructions; drain well.
2. Melt 1 tablespoon butter in a large skillet over medium high heat. Season chicken with Italian seasoning, salt and pepper, to taste. Add chicken to the skillet and cook, flipping once, until cooked through, about 3-4 minutes per side. Let cool before slicing; set aside.
3. Melt remaining 3 tablespoons butter in the skillet. Add garlic, and cook, stirring frequently, until fragrant, about 1-2 minutes. Whisk in flour, tomato paste and basil until lightly browned, about 1 minute.
4. Gradually whisk in milk and sun-dried tomatoes. Cook, whisking constantly, until slightly thickened, about 5 minutes. Stir in cream cheese and Parmesan until smooth, about 1-2 minutes. If the mixture is too thick, add more milk as needed; season with salt and pepper, to taste.
5. Stir in pasta and chicken, and gently toss to combine.
6. Serve immediately, garnished with Parmesan and parsley, if desired.

Prep Time: 10 Minutes

Cook Time: 35 Minutes

Servings: 4

Ingredients

- 4 boneless, skinless chicken breasts
- Kosher salt and freshly ground black pepper, to taste
- 1 tablespoon olive oil
- 3 cloves garlic, minced
- 1 red onion, diced
- 1 mango, diced
- ½ cup mango nectar
- 1 tablespoon freshly grated ginger
- 1 ½ teaspoons sambal oelek, ground fresh chile paste
- Juice of 1 lime
- 2 tablespoons chopped fresh cilantro leaves

For The Coconut Brown Rice:

- 1 cup brown rice
- ¼ cup coconut milk

Instructions

1. In a large saucepan filled with 2 cups of water, cook rice according to package instructions; set aside. Stir in coconut milk; set aside.
2. Season chicken with salt and pepper, to taste.
3. Preheat grill to medium high heat. Add chicken to grill and cook, flipping once until cooked through, about 5-6 minutes on each side; set aside.
4. Heat olive oil in a medium skillet over medium heat. Add garlic and onion, and cook, stirring often, until onions have become translucent, about 3-4 minutes. Stir in mango, mango nectar, ginger, sambal oelek and 1/2 cup water until slightly thickened, about 3-5 minutes. Stir in lime juice.
5. Divide rice into bowls. Top with chicken and mango mixture.
6. Serve immediately, garnished with cilantro, if desired.

Prep Time: 20 Minutes

Cook Time: 45 Minutes

Servings: 12

Ingredients

- 9 whole-wheat lasagna noodles
- 1 tablespoon olive oil
- 2 cloves garlic, minced
- 1 onion, diced
- 2 zucchinis, diced
- 1 carrot, peeled and diced
- 12 ounces ground turkey
- Salt and freshly ground black pepper, to taste
- 1 (28-ounce) can crushed tomatoes
- 1 (6-ounce) can tomato paste
- 1 tablespoon Italian seasoning
- 1 (15-ounce) package reduced-fat ricotta
- 1 (10-ounce) package frozen chopped spinach, thawed and drained
- 1/4 cup freshly grated Parmesan
- 1 large egg, beaten

- 2 1/2 cups reduced-fat shredded mozzarella
- 2 tablespoons chopped fresh parsley leaves

Instructions

1. Preheat oven to 350 degrees F. Lightly oil a 9×13 baking dish or coat with nonstick spray.
2. In a large pot of boiling salted water, cook lasagna noodles according to package instructions.
3. Heat olive oil in a large skillet over medium high heat. Add garlic, onion, zucchinis and carrot. Cook, stirring occasionally, until tender, about 3-4 minutes.
4. Stir in ground turkey and cook until turkey has browned, about 3-5 minutes, making sure to crumble the turkey as it cooks; season with salt and pepper, to taste. Drain excess fat.
5. Stir in tomatoes, tomato paste and Italian seasoning until well combined; bring to a simmer until thickened, about 8-10 minutes.
6. In a medium bowl, combine ricotta, spinach, Parmesan and egg; set aside.
7. Spread 1 cup tomato mixture onto the bottom of a 9×13 baking dish; top with 3 lasagna noodles, 1/2 of the ricotta cheese mixture and 1 cup mozzarella

cheese. Repeat with a second layer. Top with remaining noodles, tomato mixture and remaining 1/2 cup mozzarella cheese.

8. Place into oven and bake for 35-45 minutes, or until bubbling. Then broil for 2-3 minutes, or until top is browned in spots.

9. Let cool 15 minutes. Serve, garnished with parsley, if desired.

Prep Time: 15 Minutes

Cook Time: 25 Minutes

Servings: 8

Ingredients

- 1 tablespoon olive oil
- 1 pound ground beef
- 1 onion, diced
- 2 cloves garlic, minced
- 1 1.25-ounce package taco seasoning
- 1 cup rice
- 1 cup vegetable broth
- 1 15-ounce can black beans, drained and rinsed
- 1 10-ounce can Ro Mild Diced Tomatoes & Green Chilies
- 1 cup corn kernels, frozen, canned or roasted
- 1 teaspoon chili powder
- ½ teaspoon cumin
- salt and freshly ground black pepper, to taste
- Juice of 1 lime
- 2 tablespoons chopped fresh cilantro leaves

- 1 ½ cups shredded cheddar cheese
- ½ cup shredded Monterey Jack cheese
- 1 Roma tomato, diced

Instructions

1. Heat olive oil in a large skillet over medium high heat. Add ground beef, onion and garlic. Cook until beef has browned, about 3-5 minutes, making sure to crumble the beef as it cooks; stir in taco seasoning. Drain excess fat.
2. Stir in rice, vegetable broth, beans, Ro*Tel®, corn, chili powder and cumin; season with salt and pepper, to taste. Bring to a boil; cover, reduce heat and simmer until rice is cooked through, about 16-18 minutes. Stir in lime juice and cilantro.
3. Remove from heat and top with cheeses. Cover until cheese has melted, about 2 minutes.
4. Serve immediately, garnished with tomato, if desired.

Prep Time: 10 Minutes

Cook Time: 20 Minutes

Servings: 4

Ingredients

- 2 tablespoons balsamic vinegar
- 1 tablespoon honey
- 1 tablespoon olive oil
- 2 cloves garlic, minced
- salt and freshly ground black pepper, to taste
- 2 pounds brussels sprouts, halved
- 4 slices bacon, diced

For The Eggs:

- 4 large eggs
- 2 tablespoons freshly grated Parmesan
- ¼ teaspoon crushed red pepper flakes, or more, to taste
- salt and freshly ground black pepper, to taste
- 2 tablespoons chopped fresh chives

Instructions

1. Preheat oven to 400 degrees F. Lightly oil a baking sheet or coat with nonstick spray.
2. In a small bowl, whisk together balsamic vinegar, honey, olive oil and garlic; season with salt and pepper, to taste.
3. Place brussels sprouts and bacon in a single layer onto the prepared baking sheet. Stir in balsamic vinegar mixture.
4. Place into oven and bake for 10-12 minutes, or until tender.
5. Remove from oven and create 4 wells, gently cracking the eggs throughout and keeping the yolk intact.
6. Sprinkle eggs with Parmesan and red pepper flakes; season with salt and pepper, to taste.
7. Place into oven and bake until the egg whites have set, an additional 7-9 minutes.
8. Serve immediately, garnished with chives, if desired.

Prep Time: 10 Minutes

Cook Time: 50 Minutes

Servings: 6

Ingredients

- 1 tablespoon olive oil
- 2 cloves garlic, minced
- 1 onion, diced
- 1 pound cremini mushrooms, thinly sliced
- 2 teaspoons Worcestershire sauce
- ½ teaspoon dried thyme
- Kosher salt and freshly ground black pepper, to taste
- ¾ cup brown rice
- 1 ½ cups vegetable broth
- 2 tablespoons unsalted butter
- 2 tablespoons chopped fresh chives

Instructions

1. Heat olive oil in a large stockpot or Dutch oven over medium heat. Add garlic and onion, and cook, stirring frequently, until translucent, about 2-3 minutes.
2. Stir in mushrooms, Worcestershire and thyme and cook, stirring occasionally, until mushrooms are tender and browned, about 5-6 minutes; season with salt and pepper, to taste.
3. Stir in brown rice and vegetable broth. Bring to a boil; cover, reduce heat and simmer until rice is cooked through, about 40-45 minutes. Stir in butter until melted, about 1 minute.
4. Serve immediately, garnished with chives, if desired.

Prep Time: 20 Minutes

Cook Time: 20 Minutes

Servings: 4

Ingredients

- 2 tablespoons olive oil, divided
- 3 cloves garlic, minced
- 1 onion, diced
- 3 carrots, peeled and diced
- 2 stalks celery, diced
- ½ teaspoon dried thyme
- 5 cups chicken stock
- 2 bay leaves
- 2 cups baby spinach
- ¼ cup freshly grated Parmesan cheese
- 2 tablespoons chopped fresh parsley leaves

For The Meatballs:

- 1 pound ground turkey
- ⅓ cup Panko
- ¼ cup freshly grated Parmesan cheese

- ½ teaspoon dried oregano
- ½ teaspoon dried basil
- ½ teaspoon dried parsley
- ¼ teaspoon garlic powder
- ¼ teaspoon crushed red pepper flakes
- salt and freshly ground black pepper, to taste

Instructions

1. In a large bowl, combine ground turkey, Panko, Parmesan, oregano, basil, parsley, garlic powder and red pepper flakes; season with salt and pepper, to taste. Using a wooden spoon or clean hands, stir until well combined. Roll the mixture into 1 1/4-to-1 1/2-inch meatballs, forming about 18-20 meatballs.

2. Heat 1 tablespoon olive oil in a large stockpot or Dutch oven over medium heat. Add meatballs, in batches, and cook until all sides are browned, about 2-3 minutes. Transfer to a paper towel-lined plate; set aside.

3. Add remaining 1 tablespoon olive oil to the skillet. Add garlic, onion, carrots and celery. Cook, stirring occasionally, until tender, about 3-4 minutes. Stir in thyme until fragrant, about 1 minute.

4. Whisk in chicken stock, bay leaves and 1 cup water; bring to a boil. Stir in meatballs; reduce heat and simmer until meatballs are cooked through, about 10-12 minutes. Stir in spinach until wilted, about 2 minutes.
5. Serve immediately, sprinkled with Parmesan and garnished with parsley, if desired.

Prep Time: 10 Minutes

Cook Time: 25 Minutes

Servings: 6

Ingredients

- 2 teaspoons olive oil
- ¼ cup Panko
- 8 ounces PHILADELPHIA Cream Cheese, at room temperature
- 2 ½ cups fresh broccoli florets
- ¾ cup shredded cheddar cheese, divided
- ½ cup sour cream
- ¼ cup grated Parmesan
- ¼ cup milk
- 1 tablespoon Emeril's Essence Creole Seasoning
- ½ teaspoon garlic powder
- ½ teaspoon onion powder
- salt and freshly ground black pepper, to taste

Instructions

1. Preheat oven to 375 degrees F. Lightly oil a 9-inch baking dish or coat with nonstick spray.
2. Heat olive oil in a large skillet over medium high heat. Add Panko and cook, stirring, until browned and toasted, about 3 minutes; set aside.
3. In a large bowl, combine cream cheese, broccoli, 1/2 cup cheddar cheese, sour cream, Parmesan, milk, Emeril's Essence, garlic powder and onion powder; season with salt and pepper, to taste.
4. Spread broccoli mixture into the prepared baking dish; sprinkle with remaining 1/4 cup cheddar cheese. Place into oven and bake until bubbly, about 20-25 minutes.
5. Serve immediately, sprinkled with Panko, if desired.

Prep Time: 10 Minutes

Cook Time: 20 Minutes

Servings: 4

Ingredients

- 1 pound spaghetti
- 2 tablespoons vegetable oil
- 3 boneless, skinless thin-sliced chicken breasts
- Kosher salt and freshly ground black pepper, to taste
- 4 cloves garlic, minced
- ½ cup dry roasted peanuts
- 2 green onions, thinly sliced

For The Sauce:

- ½ cup reduced sodium soy sauce
- ½ cup chicken broth
- ½ cup dry sherry
- 2 tablespoons red chili paste with garlic, or more, to taste
- ¼ cup sugar
- 2 tablespoons red wine vinegar

- 2 tablespoons cornstarch
- 1 tablespoon sesame oil

Instructions

1. In a small bowl, whisk together soy sauce, chicken broth, dry sherry, red chili paste, sugar, red wine vinegar, cornstarch and sesame oil; set aside.
2. In a large pot of boiling salted water, cook pasta according to package instructions; drain well.
3. Heat vegetable oil in a large skillet over medium high heat. Season chicken breasts with salt and pepper, to taste. Add to skillet and cook, flipping once, until cooked through, about 3-4 minutes per side. Let cool before dicing into bite-size pieces; set aside.
4. Add garlic to the skillet and cook, stirring constantly, until fragrant, about 1 minute. Stir in soy sauce mixture and bring to a boil; reduce heat and simmer until thickened, about 1-2 minutes. Stir in pasta, chicken, peanuts and green onions.
5. Serve immediately.

21. Enchilada Pasta

Prep Time: 10 Minutes

Cook Time: 20 Minutes

Servings: 4

Ingredients

- 16 ounces extra wide egg noodles
- 1 ¼ cups enchilada sauce
- 1 cup canned corn kernels, drained
- 1 cup canned black beans, drained and rinsed
- 1 cup shredded cheddar cheese, divided
- 1 cup shredded Monterey Jack cheese, divided
- ¼ cup Greek yogurt
- 1 4-ounce can diced green chiles
- 1 tablespoon olive oil
- 1 pound ground beef
- 4 ounces cream cheese
- ½ teaspoon chili powder, or more to taste
- ¼ teaspoon cumin
- salt and freshly ground black pepper, to taste

- 1 avocado, halved, seeded, peeled and diced
- 2 tablespoons chopped fresh cilantro leaves

Instructions

1. Preheat oven to 350 degrees F. Lightly oil a 9×13 baking dish or coat with nonstick spray.
2. In a large pot of boiling salted water, cook pasta according to package instructions; drain well.
3. In a large bowl, combine enchilada sauce, corn, beans, 1/2 cup cheddar cheese, 1/2 cup Monterey Jack cheese, Greek yogurt and green chiles; set aside.
4. Heat olive oil in a saucepan over medium high heat. Add ground beef and cook until browned, about 3-5 minutes, making sure to crumble the beef as it cooks; drain excess fat.
5. Stir in cream cheese, chili powder and cumin until cream cheese has melted. Stir in pasta and enchilada mixture until well combined; season with salt and pepper, to taste.
6. Add pasta to prepared baking dish and top with avocado and remaining cheeses. Place into oven and bake until cheeses have melted, about 5-10 minutes.
7. Serve immediately, garnished with cilantro.

Prep Time: 10 Minutes

Cook Time: 40 Minutes

Servings: 4

Ingredients

- 2 tablespoons unsalted butter
- 1 large leek, thinly sliced
- 1 large red bell pepper, diced
- 2 cups milk
- 3 tablespoons all-purpose flour
- 3 cups vegetable broth
- 2 cups roasted corn kernels
- 2 pounds red potatoes, cubed
- 1 ½ teaspoons Emeril's Essence Creole Seasoning
- ¾ teaspoon thyme
- ¾ teaspoon salt
- Chopped fresh chives, for garnish

For Emeril's Essence Creole Seasoning:

- 2 ½ tablespoons paprika
- 2 tablespoons garlic powder

- 2 tablespoons salt
- 1 tablespoon onion powder
- 1 tablespoon cayenne pepper
- 1 tablespoon oregano
- 1 tablespoon thyme
- 1 tablespoon black pepper

Instructions

1. To make Emeril's Essence, combine paprika, garlic powder, salt, onion powder, cayenne pepper, oregano, thyme and pepper; set aside.
2. Melt butter in a large stockpot or Dutch oven over medium heat. Add leeks and bell pepper, and cook, stirring occasionally, until tender, about 5 minutes. Gradually whisk in milk and flour, and cook, whisking constantly, until incorporated, about 1-2 minutes. Stir in vegetable broth, corn kernels, potatoes, 1 1/2 teaspoons Emeril's Essence, thyme and salt.
3. Bring to a boil; reduce heat and simmer until potatoes are tender, about 20-30 minutes.
4. Serve immediately, garnished with chives.

Prep Time: 10 Minutes

Cook Time: 20 Minutes

Servings: 4

Ingredients

- 1 pound flank steak, thinly sliced across the grain
- ¼ cup cornstarch
- ½ cup vegetable oil
- 2 green onions, thinly sliced

For The Sauce:

- ¼ cup reduced sodium soy sauce
- ½ cup brown sugar, packed
- 3 cloves garlic, minced
- 2 teaspoons grated fresh ginger
- 2 teaspoons vegetable oil

Instructions

1. In a medium bowl, whisk together soy sauce, brown sugar, garlic, ginger, 2 teaspoons vegetable oil and 1/2

cup water. Heat soy sauce mixture in a medium saucepan until slightly thickened, about 5-10 minutes; set aside.

2. In a large bowl, combine flank steak and cornstarch.

3. Heat 1/2 cup vegetable oil in a large saucepan. Add beef and fry until browned and cooked through, about 1-2 minutes. Transfer to a paper towel-lined plate; discard excess oil.

4. Add beef and soy sauce mixture to the saucepan over medium heat and cook until sauce thickens, about 2-3 minutes. Stir in green onions.

5. Serve immediately.

Prep Time: 20 Minutes

Cook Time: 25 Minutes

Servings: 4

Ingredients

For The Ham:

- 2 tablespoons apricot preserves
- 1 teaspoon Dijon mustard
- 1 teaspoon apple cider vinegar
- ½ teaspoon finely chopped fresh rosemary
- salt and freshly ground pepper, to taste
- 3 8-ounce ham steaks

For The Sweet Potatoes:

- 6 small to medium sweet potatoes
- 3 tablespoons unsalted butter, cubed
- 1 ½ cups mini marshmallows
- ½ cup candied pecans, chopped

For The Green Beans:

- 1 pound green beans, trimmed

- 1 ½ tablespoons olive oil

- 2 cloves garlic, minced

- salt and freshly ground black pepper, to taste

For The Biscuits (Optional):

- Flaky Mile High Biscuits

Instructions

1. Preheat oven to 400 degrees F. Lightly oil two baking sheets or coat with nonstick spray.

For The Ham:

2. In a small bowl, whisk together apricot preserves, Dijon, vinegar and rosemary; season with salt and pepper, to taste.
3. Place ham steaks onto one side of the prepared baking sheet, slightly overlapping. Brush evenly with apricot preserves mixture.

For The Sweet Potatoes:

1. Pierce sweet potatoes with a fork; place into microwave for 8-10 minutes, or until tender. Cut the potatoes down the center lengthwise, top with butter, marshmallows and pecans.

2. Place sweet potatoes onto the opposite side of the ham steaks in a single layer.

For The Green Beans:

1. Place green beans in a single layer onto the second prepared baking sheet. Add olive oil and garlic; season with salt and pepper to taste. Gently toss to combine.
2. Place into oven and bake until the marshmallows just start to brown and the green beans are tender, about 20-25 minutes. Add biscuits during the last 3-5 minutes of cooking time, if desired.
3. Serve immediately.

Prep Time: 15 Minutes

Cook Time: 15 Minutes

Servings: 4

Ingredients

- 4 (6-ounce) salmon fillets
- Salt and freshly ground black pepper, to taste
- 1 ½ tablespoons unsalted butter
- 2 cloves garlic, minced
- 1 medium shallot, diced
- 2 tablespoons all-purpose flour
- ¼ cup dry white wine
- ¾ cup chicken stock
- ¾ cup half and half
- 3 cups baby spinach
- 2 tablespoons chopped fresh dill
- 1 lemon, cut in wedges

Instructions

1. Using paper towels, pat both sides of the salmon fillets dry; season with 1 teaspoon salt and 1/2 teaspoon pepper.
2. Melt butter in a large cast iron skillet over medium heat. Add salmon fillets to the skillet, skin side up, and cook until golden brown and a crust has formed, about 4-5 minutes. Using a fish turner, flip, and cook for an additional 4-5 minutes, or until desired doneness. Remove and keep warm.
3. Reduce heat to low; add garlic and shallots, and cook, stirring frequently, until fragrant, about 2 minutes.
4. Whisk in flour until lightly browned, about 1 minute.
5. Stir in wine, scraping any browned bits from the bottom of the skillet.
6. Stir in chicken stock and half and half until slightly thickened, about 2-3 minutes; season with salt and pepper, to taste.
7. Stir in spinach until wilted, about 1-2 minutes. Return salmon to the skillet; sprinkle with dill.
8. Serve immediately with lemon wedges.

Prep Time: 15 Minutes

Cook Time: 25 Minutes

Servings: 6

Ingredients

- 2 tablespoons olive oil
- ¼ cup yellow cornmeal
- 1 pound pizza dough, homemade or store-bought
- ½ cup plus 2 tablespoons favorite bbq sauce, we love Stubb's
- 2 cups leftover shredded rotisserie chicken
- 1 cup shredded smoked cheddar cheese
- 1 cup shredded whole milk mozzarella cheese
- ½ cup diced red onion
- Kosher salt and freshly ground pepper, to taste
- 3 tablespoons chopped fresh cilantro leaves

Instructions

1. Preheat oven to 450 degrees F. Lightly coat a baking sheet or pizza pan with olive oil.

2. Working on a surface that has been sprinkled with cornmeal, roll out the pizza into a 12-inch-diameter round. Transfer to prepared baking sheet or pizza pan.

3. Using a small ladle, spread bbq sauce over the surface of the dough in an even layer, leaving a 1/2-inch border.

4. Top with chicken, cheeses and onion; season with salt and pepper, to taste.

5. Place into oven and bake for 20-24 minutes, or until the crust is golden brown and the cheeses have melted.

6. Serve immediately, garnished with cilantro, if desired.

Prep Time: 10 Minutes

Cook Time: 10 Minutes

Servings: 4

Ingredients

- 8 tablespoons unsalted butter, cubed and divided
- 4 cloves garlic, minced
- 1 medium shallot, minced
- 1 ½ teaspoons chili powder
- ½ teaspoon smoked paprika
- 1 pound medium shrimp, peeled and deveined
- Kosher salt and freshly ground black pepper, to taste
- ⅓ cup vegetable or chicken stock
- 2 tablespoons honey
- 1 tablespoon freshly squeezed lime juice
- 2 teaspoons lime zest
- 2 tablespoons chopped fresh cilantro leaves

Instructions

1. Melt 6 tablespoons butter in a large skillet over medium heat.
2. Add garlic and shallot, and cook, stirring frequently, until fragrant, about 1 minute. Stir in chili powder and paprika.
3. Add shrimp; season with salt and pepper, to taste. Cook, stirring occasionally, until pink and cooked through, about 3-4 minutes.
4. Stir in vegetable or chicken stock, honey, lime juice and lime zest, scraping any browned bits from the bottom of the skillet.
5. Remove from heat; stir in cilantro and remaining 2 tablespoons butter until melted.
6. Serve immediately.

Prep Time: 30 Minutes

Cook Time: 6hrs 10 Minutes

Servings: 8

Ingredients

- 1 4 1/2 pound center-cut corned beef brisket, excess fat trimmed
- 3 tablespoons whole grain mustard
- ¼ teaspoon ground allspice
- ¼ teaspoon ground cloves
- Kosher salt and freshly ground black pepper, to taste
- 1 medium sweet onion, sliced
- 1 head cabbage, cut into 2-inch wedges
- 3 tablespoons olive oil, divided
- 2 pounds medium red potatoes, quartered
- 3 large carrots, cut into 3-inch pieces
- 2 tablespoons chopped fresh parsley leaves

Instructions

1. Place corned beef in a large bowl and cover with cold water; let stand 1-2 hours. Rinse with cold water and thoroughly pat dry.
2. Preheat oven to 325 degrees F. Line a 9x13 baking dish with foil.

Mustard Mixture:

1. In a small bowl, combine mustard, allspice, cloves and 1 teaspoon pepper.
2. Place corned beef onto the prepared baking dish. Spread MUSTARD MIXTURE evenly over one side of the corned beef; top with onions. Fold up all 4 sides of the foil over the corned beef, covering completely and sealing the packet closed.
3. Place into oven and bake until tender, about 3 1/2-4 hours; let stand covered.
4. Increase oven temperature to 425 degrees F. Line two baking sheets with parchment paper.
5. Brush cabbage with 1 tablespoon olive oil. Place in a single layer onto the prepared baking sheet; season with salt and pepper, to taste.
6. Place potatoes and carrots in a single layer onto the second prepared baking sheet. Add remaining 2

tablespoons olive oil; gently toss to combine. Season
with salt and pepper, to taste.

7. Place sheet pans into oven, on separate racks, and
   bake until cabbage is lightly charred and potatoes and
   carrots are tender, about 30-35 minutes, rotating pans
   and stirring halfway through baking.

8. Thinly slice corned beef against the grain and serve
   with onions, cabbage, potatoes and carrots, garnished
   with parsley, if desired.

Prep Time: 20 Minutes

Cook Time: 20 Minutes

Servings: 4

Ingredients

- 1 ½ teaspoons chili powder
- 2 teaspoons ground cumin
- 2 teaspoons dried oregano
- 1 teaspoon smoked paprika
- Kosher salt and freshly ground black pepper, to taste
- 1 red bell pepper, cut into strips
- 1 yellow bell pepper, cut into strips
- 1 orange bell pepper, cut into strips
- 1 sweet onion, cut into wedges
- 3 cloves garlic, minced
- 3 tablespoons olive oil, divided
- 1 ½ pounds medium shrimp, peeled and deveined
- ¼ cup chopped fresh cilantro leaves
- 1 tablespoon freshly squeezed lime juice
- 6 8-inch flour or corn tortillas, warmed

Instructions

1. Preheat oven to 425 degrees F. Lightly oil a baking sheet or coat with nonstick spray.

Chili Powder Mixture:

2. In a small bowl, combine chili powder, cumin, oregano, paprika, 1 teaspoon salt and 1 teaspoon pepper.
3. Place bell peppers, onion and garlic in a single layer onto the prepared baking sheet. Stir in 2 tablespoons olive oil and half the CHILI POWDER MIXTURE; gently toss to combine.
4. Place into oven and bake for 10 minutes, or until the vegetables are beginning to soften.
5. In a large bowl, combine shrimp and remaining 1 tablespoon olive oil and CHILI Powder Mixture.
6. Working carefully, move vegetables onto one side of the baking sheet. Place shrimp onto the opposite side of the baking sheet in a single layer.
7. Place into oven and bake just until shrimp are pink, firm and cooked through, an additional 6-8 minutes. Stir in cilantro and lime juice.
8. Serve immediately with tortillas.

Prep Time: 45 Minutes

Cook Time: 1hrs 20 Minutes

Servings: 4

Ingredients

For The Stuffing/Dressing

- 10 cups brioche bread cubes
- 3 tablespoons unsalted butter
- ½ medium sweet onion, diced
- 2 celebry ribs, diced
- ¼ cup dry white wine
- 3 tablespoons chopped fresh parley leaves
- 1 tablespoon chopped fresh sage leaves
- 1 tablespoon chopped fresh thyme leaves
- Kosher salt and freshly ground black pepper, to taste
- 1 ¼ cups chicken stock

For The Turkey:

- 3 tablespoons unsalted butter, at room temperature
- 1 ½ tablespoons chopped fresh parley leaves
- 2 teaspoons poultry seasoning

- 2 cloves garlic, minced

- Kosher salt and freshly ground black pepper, to taste

- 1 2-pound skin-on, boneless turkey breast

For The Brussels Sprouts:

- 1 ½ pounds brussels sprouts, halved

- 1 ½ tablespoons olive oil

- 1 ½ tablespoons reduced sodium soy sauce

- 1 tablespoon honey

For The Sweet Potatoes:

- 6 small to medium sweet potatoes

- 3 tablespoons unsalted butter, cubed

- 1 ½ cups mini marshmallows

- ½ cup candied pecans, chopped

Instructions

1. Preheat oven to 425 degrees F. Lightly oil two baking sheets or coat with nonstick spray.

For The Stuffing/Dressing:

1. Spread bread cubes in a single layer onto the prepared baking sheet. Place into oven and bake until crisp and golden, about 10-12 minutes; set aside.

2. Melt butter in a large Dutch oven over medium-high heat. Add onion and celery, and cook, stirring occasionally, until tender, about 3-4 minutes.

3. Stir in wine and cook, stirring occasionally, until just reduced, about 2 minutes. Stir in parsley, sage and thyme. Remove from heat and stir in bread; season with salt and pepper, to taste. Stir in chicken stock until absorbed and well combined. Place bread mixture onto one side of the prepared baking sheet in a single layer.

For The Turkey:

1. In a small bowl, combine butter, parsley, poultry seasoning, garlic, 3/4 teaspoon salt and 1/2 teaspoon pepper. Using your fingers, carefully loosen the skin from the breast meat, spreading the butter mixture under the skin. Secure skin over the butter with wooden picks; season with salt and pepper, to taste. Place onto the opposite side of the prepared baking sheet.

For The Brussels Sprouts:

1. Place brussels sprouts in a single layer onto the second prepared baking sheet. Add olive oil, soy sauce and honey; gently toss to combine.

For The Sweet Potatoes:

1. Pierce sweet potatoes with a fork; place into microwave for 8-10 minutes, or until tender. Cut the potatoes down the center lengthwise, top with butter, marshmallows and pecans.
2. Place sheet pans into oven, on separate racks, and bake for 20 minutes. Remove from oven; stir brussels sprouts and rotate sheet pans onto different racks. Continue to bake until brussels sprouts are lightly browned, an additional 10 minutes. Stir brussels sprouts onto one side of the baking sheet.
3. Place sweet potatoes onto the opposite side of the brussels sprouts in a single layer. Place into oven and bake until the marshmallows just start to brown, about 5 minutes.
4. Continue cooking the turkey and stuffing until the turkey is completely cooked through, reaching an internal temperature of 165 degrees F, an additional 20-25 minutes. Let rest 5 minutes before slicing.
5. Serve immediately.

www.ingramcontent.com/pod-product-compliance
Lightning Source LLC
Chambersburg PA
CBHW050050260726
48658CB00005B/1864